I0476685

The
TRUTH
About What Is
In *Your*
Medicine
Cabinet...

What Is Medication
Safety?

by Vanessa LeSure-Walker

Copyright © 2015 by Vanessa Walker.

All rights reserved. No part of this publication may be reproduced, distributed, or transmitted in any form or by any means, including photocopying, recording, or other electronic or mechanical methods, without the prior written permission of the publisher, except in the case of brief quotations embodied in critical reviews and certain other noncommercial uses permitted by copyright law. For permission requests, write to the publisher, addressed "Attention: Permissions Coordinator," at the address below.

Author: Vanessa LeSure-Walker

www.theaphtiproject.com

The APhTI Project/ Vanessa Walker.—1st ed.
ISBN-13:
978-1514185254

ISBN-10:
1514185253

The information in this book is not intended to take the place of your prescriber and your pharmacist. This book is intended to start a dialogue between practitioners and patient on an individual level and on a corporate level.

FOREWORD

If you picked up this book, you have made a great choice. Many times when we ask questions about the medications we are prescribed or the ones we purchase over the counter, we are met with lots of words that we do not understand and end up being more confused than when we first got the notion to ask the question.

When Vanessa contacted me to write the foreword for this book, I was happy to do it for two reasons. The first is that she is a friend of mine who I have seen talk about her mission and her passion for Pharmacy Technicians and for Medication Safety.

The second is that I believe that this book will become a wonderful go to reference for those who want to become more savvy about Medication Safety.

The TRUTH About What Is In Your Medicine Cabinet: What Is Medication Safety? is packed with information in a conversational tone and filled with tips and tools that have come directly from the thoughts and understandings of an experienced Pharmacist and Trainer. I'm sure that you will be glad you made the purchase.

JoAnn Youngblood King, Success Coach, Speaker, Business Trainer
www.liveyourpotential.com

ACKNOWLEDGMENTS

To my Lord and Savior Jesus Christ, who makes all things possible and without Him everything becomes impossible.

To Dorothy and James, who raised me, nurtured me and guided me.

To Curtis Walker, with love and affection . . .

To James Jr, much love!

To my children, greater than this is possible for you—BELIEVE!

The

TRUTH

About What Is In Your Medicine Cabinet...

What Is Medication Safety?

Vanessa LeSure-Walker, RPh

Table of Contents

INTRODUCTION

I have wanted to tell people these things for a long time and struggled with whether or not I had an audience who would listen.

Looking back, my fondest times in the pharmacy were when I got to speak to people and help them work through their medication issues. The times that gave me the most joy in the classroom was seeing the eyes of the student at the pivotal moment between confusion and understanding and knowing that I somehow had a hand in the process. It's at times like these when I could feel the hand of God with me and I have become unstoppable because of it.

It is my hope that you learn from this book but even more that you enjoy reading it as much as I enjoyed putting it together for YOU!

PART OF MY STORY

So this book is about medication safety. The easiest way that I can translate to you my passion about this topic is to tell you a story. This may seem like another author that is telling you their story but *this* story is different. Not just because it happened to me but because it could happen to you! It could happen to anyone actually. So this story although it is my story, is *our* story. The fact that I have the education that I have only makes this story harder for me to tell because the fact that this happened to me caused me a lot of guilt for many years.

As a pharmacist, I have been taught to analyze problems and come up with solutions. In my career, that is one of the things that I did every day for countless numbers of other people. When the situation that I am going to chronicle here happened, my first emotion was bewilderment and my second emotion was guilt. When I say that the guilt lasted for years, that would not be far from the truth...

I have shared pieces of this story before now, in my own classroom. Now I am telling the world, so that someone can learn from my experience and not have to repeat my mistake. By now, you must be wondering what could this story be? Well, let me tell you about it!

It was about 20 years ago, which would make it sometime in the summer of a year in the mid 1990's. At the time, I was a Pharmacist with less than five years under my belt. It was that "in between time." You know the time in a person's career when they have not spent enough time in a profession to be called seasoned but they have worked enough in their industry not to be called a newbie. Well, that's where I was professionally.

My parents had a Brownstone in the Brooklyn area and so in order to help them with the bills, I stayed in one of the apartments that they would normally rent to someone else. My mother was a long time asthmatic and to make matters worse, she had a litany of allergies. I am not talking one or two here but about twenty. She was allergic to common things like corn and apples and some things not so common like horse serum (this made getting certain vaccinations not feasible for her).

My mother had suffered with asthma for about forty years and was often in the hospital to get treatments for her condition. She was the type of person who took everything in stride even to the point of borderline secrecy especially when it came to her health.

My mom would sometimes have attacks in the middle of the night and she would get up and go to the hospital on her own. She would not even tell my dad that she was going and we would all find out about it the following day. Of course, we would always read her the riot act and she would respond with, " I'm fine".

But one day, she was not fine. She had taken a cab to the emergency room but blacked out in the cab. She had no recollection of getting out of the cab, all she knew is that four days later, she was in the ICU.

My mother had suffered a stroke! When I arrived at the hospital to see her, she was not conscious. Although she could not see me, what I saw was every tube that she was connected to. I saw that she had to be intubated (she had a breathing tube and was on a respirator) , I saw that her heart rate was being closely monitored, I saw the blood in her hair, I saw everything and as I cried, J prayed to God and asked Him to heal my mother and to not let her die. I knew that this event was related to her fight with asthma. I also knew that everything would now change!

My mother regained consciousness and for three days she was blind. It was weird for me to see my mom who was always so full of life, hope and optimistic about everything in that state. Thankfully, her sight did return but she had a difficult road ahead. She had to spend a few weeks in a rehab facility where she had to learn how to use her limbs again. Mom lived for a good ten years after that incident with no real visible signs of what had happened! That is a miracle from God!

What I found out during our conversations after my mom's stroke is that my mother had been overusing her asthma pump and had gone through one pump and part of another one in less than a month. I knew that that was way too much and it was then that I understood. Despite the numerous conversations that we had about asthma, she did not fully understand her medication and the side effects or what could happen in an overdose situation. She had inadvertently overdosed herself and wound up in the hospital because of it.

We have all heard that a little knowledge is dangerous and this is a prime example of that.

So, I have had a very personal introduction to medication safety and what could happen to people that are ignorant of it or ignore it.

You see your medication is an tool like a hammer; and like a hammer, it's use can be either constructive or destructive. When dealing with medications, there are some things that you must know:

Medications are classified as drugs and the word "drug" is a legal word. All legal words have legal definitions. Lay people say "medication" but practitioners say "drugs".

What is a drug? Before I get to that, let me say that we call many substances drugs, even when they are not. A person, company or entity, etc., cannot call their product a drug unless they have approval to do so from the FDA. They also cannot say that their product lines up with any of the parts of the definition of the word drug.

Let me draw a parallel. If I say that I am going to eat a chocolate chip cookie, I have stated to you exactly what I will consume. But what if I say the following statement to you? I am going to eat a flat pastry that is round and has bits of chocolate in it, in your mind you will more than likely picture a cookie. So a person cannot say a product is a drug or say a product has the attributes of a drug without getting the FDA's approval.

So what is a drug? As per the FDA's, Food and Drug Administration, this is the 3 part definition.

1.   any substance that is recognized in one of these references: the United States Pharmacopeia, the National Formulary, or the Homeopathic Pharmacopeia of the United States.
2.   something intended for use in diagnosis, pure mitigation, treatment or prevention of disease in man or animals.
3.   something other than food intended to affect the structure or any function of the body of man or animals.

There is not a drug in existence that has no side effect(s). So every drug has at least one side effect.

 Some negative effects are bearable and some aren't. Some are downright deadly. In medicine, this is called "Risk vs Benefit". In other words, if the benefits far outweigh the risks, we see value in continuing that therapy.

If it is the other way around and the risks outweigh the benefits, there is less value placed in starting or continuing that therapy. Who uses risk vs benefit? Everyone! If you know that a drug that you are taking has an undesirable side effect, would you still take it? It probably depends on what you are taking it for. Are you managing the discomfort of a cold or are you being treated for cancer?

Unless it is life and death...if a medication is less than five years old, you should carefully consider your options before taking it.

To help you understand why I say this, I am going to draw a parallel to something completely unrelated to medicine. You know that we live in a world of gadgets and anytime a new gadget or a new version of an old gadget is about to hit the market, there is always a lot of buzz. There are advertising campaigns, so many that we get tired of them. I have found myself just wishing that the company involved would just release the gadget, so we can stop hearing about it.

People wait in line for days to be the first to get the new gizmo and finally the masses are able to have this long awaited thing. Once the gadget is owned by the elite few, we start to hear about the all of the negatives ranging from what the gadget does not do to how this gadget could be harmful if...

Face it the more you know about your medications, the better off you and your loved ones will be!

WHAT IS MEDICATION SAFETY?

Inherently, I believe that everyone knows what it is by knowing what it isn't. I searched and searched for a definition of what it is and came up with a blank. I don't want to say something contrite like safety with medications, although true, I don't want you to feel that you have purchased this book and all that I will say is that.

So let me start by saying there are some key areas of medication safety and if one of these areas is compromised, the medicine(aka the drug) is now unsafe. These areas are:

Prescribing

Obtaining

Using

Storing

Disposing

Reporting

I like to think that not only are these areas important for individuals but they are important for us as a society. Some of the areas, patients, their families and their caregivers have very little involvement in are prescribing and reporting. But in many instances you can shift the tides by asking the right questions.

You see due to the complex nature of our healthcare system, the onus is being placed more and more on the consumers of healthcare to be their own healthcare advocates. This shift can result in more positive outcomes if more of the consumers of healthcare have more information about its intricacies. This point brings me right back to the primary player of healthcare---drugs!

"All you do back there is count my pills and put them in a bottle, why does it take so long?" ----the unnamed customer at the Pharmacy

DON'T BE A VICTIM OF DRUG MIS-INFORMATION!

If I had a quarter for every time that I have heard someone say that all the Pharmacist has to do is count pills and put them into a bottle! I just shake my head because if the public really understood what pharmacists do and how hard we work...that negative sentiment would die fast! Let me give you some insight!

Whenever a Pharmacist gets a question from you about your medication therapy, it is important that he or she knows something about you. When I worked in the hospital setting, it was routine for us to have certain information readily at hand. We need to absolutely have information about your known allergies, we need to know other things about you such as your height and weight.

It is important for us to get as much information as possible. What you should know about your medications is that some drugs are dosed with a *standardized dosing*. What that means is that there is not a variety of doses. For most if not all situations, no matter what the individual characteristics of a person are, he or she will get the same dose and same dosing schedule as someone with different parameters. For example, there is a drug that is used to lower cholesterol named gemfibrozil (that is the drugs generic name). This drug is dosed the same way whether the person is male or female; thin or fat, elder or not. There are other drugs that are dosed with standardized dosing , not just this one.

You should also know that there are certain drugs that are dosed by the patient's weight and then sometimes height and weight together. When I think of weight there are some drugs that are dosed by a patient's actual weight and then there are some drugs that are dosed by ideal weight. Many of the antibiotics are dosed by the patients actual weight. There are some drugs that are highly toxic or cause an undesirable effect that increases when more drug is in the body. In this case, it makes more sense to have as little of that drug in the body as is necessary to obtain the desired effect.

Most practitioners believe that there should be just enough drug in the body to give the desired effect. We really don't want to give more drug than what is necessary because the adverse effects may increase with not real added benefit.

I could go on and on to tell you about the intricacies of drug dosing but that is not the only thing that drug information encompasses.

"Is the patient on any other medications?" This is a question that we Pharmacists routinely ask. We need to know if you are taking anything that may alter the way the drug written on the prescription will work. When I say the word drug here, I mean anything that will alter the patient's body. This may extend from pharmaceuticals (meaning-- prescription drugs, behind the counter drugs and over the counter drugs) to nutritional supplements to foods.

As a consumer and a patient, you must understand that there is such a thing as drug interactions. Not only do some drugs not *play* well together but some drugs and herbal remedies don't *like* to be in the same sand box either. To make things even more interesting, some foods and beverages don't mix well with medications either. That grapefruit juice that you love and is part of your daily routine is a no-no when you are taking certain drugs. Many of these drugs are used for cholesterol lowering and blood pressure maintenance.

You know, there are some drugs that it matters whether a person is male or female for proper dosing to occur. There is a class of antibiotics called the Aminoglycosides. In order for these drugs to be dosed appropriately in adults, there is one equation that is routinely used called Cockroft Gault (although the name is not as important as what I am about to share with you next). This equation has to be multiplied by 0.85 for female patients. We look at the blood levels of the drug in order to ascertain whether this drug is being dosed properly. Getting this wrong could result in serious injury to the patient. Although the aminoglycosides are used in retail, they are used topically and we don't have to worry about blood levels then. But knowing this, should make you respect your pharmacist and the things that they do behind the scenes on a daily basis to help others have a better quality of life.

There is so much more to say about drug information. I could not possibly list everything here! To truly understand it, you must become a student of it.

"I just got my package that email company in
_____ (you name the country) and
they were selling V!@gr@ and I didn't even
need a prescription." ----*Author, Poor Soul#1*

YOU DO GET YOUR MEDICINES SAFELY, DON'T YOU?

This is a situation where the red flag must have been flown at half mast. Yet, how many times have we heard of people getting their medications off the internet? I am not saying that all internet pharmacies are bad. What I am saying is do your due diligence! There are some pharmacies on the internet that are doing the right thing and there are those that are not.

You as the consumer should not get caught in the balance. There are some things that separate legitimate pharmacies on the internet from those that are illegitimate. You need to look for the VIPPS or vet-VIPPS seal or even better look for the dot pharmacy (.pharmacy) extension onto the web url.

If you get your medication from an illegal pharmacy and you are harmed because of it, what is your legal recourse? Assuming that you live to tell the tale, who do you sue for damages? The internet is everywhere and nowhere. It's reach goes into just about every home, school, library, etc but you can't go to a physical location and say this is where the internet is physically.

As a consumer, you should be aware that drug counterfeiting is big! You should want the assurance that your medicine has been obtained through legal channels and that there is a paper trail that starts at the drug's manufacturer, leads to a reputable wholesaler, goes to a dispenser or prescriber's office where you, the patient can obtain it legally!

Some of these non-legal establishments sell colored cement, rat poison and everything in between! Caveat emptor (latin for ,"let the buyer beware") applies here Be safe not sorry!

Personally, I am not a fan of Mail Order Pharmacies, either. I am old school, I think that things go better when you have a relationship with your Pharmacist. He or she knows you by name, knows your family and is in your neighborhood. Sadly, this type of relationship is becoming more and more rare. I think that the idea of the Neighborhood Pharmacist needs to be resurrected. Many of us as consumers, don't have a choice anymore when it comes to pharmacy services and I think that is a disservice to the public. Many of these pharmacies are mom and pop, independent stores that have tremendous value and provide excellent, personalized service.

Kevin had a sore throat last week and he has some of his antibiotic left over. I'm going to use it for _my_ sore throat! ---*Author, Poor Soul#2*

SAFETY IN USING MEDICATIONS

Not only do you have to be concerned about the proper dosage of medication but practitioners have to be sure that the patient receives the right drug for what is being treated. In medicine there is something called the" Rights of the Patient". In Pharmacy, we say that the patient is to receive the right drug at the right time in the right amount but we have to make sure that the drug is for the right condition.

Many people think that if one tablet works well, two tablets should work better. It sounds logical to someone that does not understand the many consequences that this way of thinking can cause.

There are some medications that when they are released into the bloodstream they are highly bound to the proteins in the blood. In this scenario, when the percentage of bound drug to free drug is altered, bad things can happen. What I am describing is a hidden way of overdosing on a medication.

You see, if a person takes two instead of one that may be an overdose because twice as much drug gets into the bloodstream. But if the percentage of a free drug in the bloodstream doubles, that also results in an overdose because twice the intended amount of drug is *free* (able) to exert an effect. What can cause something like this to happen? Well competition from another drug that is in the patient's system, can shift the balance of free drug to bound drug.

So not only is taking too much of a drug a problem but taking medication that is intended for someone else is also a problem. So much so that it violates Federal law. It is important not to self diagnose. If Jimmy has a toothache because he has a cavity, don't assume that your mouth pain is due to the same thing. Don't make your assumption worse by taking his medication. What if you are allergic to it? What if it is expired? What if he gives (accidentally of course) you the wrong medicine?

Are you beginning to see why it is important that you obtain your medication through legal channels?

Janice says,"It feels warm in here"...Phyllis says "I feel cold". Janice and Phyllis are sitting in the same room! What gives?

Safety in Storing Medication

One of the most important things to know about medications that is under your control is how to store them. Know that temperature is specific but our interpretation of the feeling of temperature is subjective. What I am saying is that what is cold to one person may not be cold to another. What is hot to one person, may not be hot to another person.

All is well and fine until we talk about the storage of medication. Manufacturers have studied the drugs that they market at length; they have to do this and have this information at the ready. So they know what temperatures are optimal to store their products. This is one very good reason why some medications require refrigeration, why some need to be frozen and why some need to be kept at room temperature.

But what are the temperatures that correspond to each one of those environments? For this, we have temperature ranges that are absolute. In order to standardize medication storage we must use the same definitions for these environments across the board. There is a reference called the USP/NF (United States Pharmacopeia and National Formulary) that gives us specific ranges for what each of these environments are temperature- wise. So what I am saying is that this reference has defined the following:

what a cold place is

what a warm place is

what a freezer is

what a refrigerator is

what room temperature is

what controlled room temperature is

what excessive heat is

The beauty in this is that there is no guesswork. This is important because when medications are kept in environments that are warmer than what is recommended, the rate at which the drug will break down increases. This means that the medication will expire sooner than what the manufacturer has stated. More boldly stated, the manufacturer's expiration date now becomes a lie!

But enough about temperature...

I am going to tell you something that is going to be very surprising to you---shocking even. You may want to sit down for this!

Most people have no clue how to store their medications and do what society dictates. They put their medications in the medicine cabinet and this is the absolute worst place to store medicine. Why?

Well, aside from temperature variances, the bathroom is where most medicine cabinets are and this area of the house is subject to lots of humidity. Humidity is not good for the stability of your medicine!

So that 10 minute hot shower that you love to take is wreaking havoc on your medicine (ask you Dermatologist, it may not be that good for your skin either).

The fact is you should store your medicine in a cool, dry place that is *secure*...

Security of your medication is also important. I'm sure that you have seen it depicted on television. One nosy person comes to a dinner party and then goes to the bathroom sometime later. While in the bathroom, "Mr Nosey" goes through the host's medicine cabinet, "just because". Usually it's a humorous depiction and the event and its aftermath usually get a good laugh from the audience.

But this can and does happen in real life! Some people will even steal your medicine from your medicine cabinet especially if it has an addiction potential at all. Unbeknownst to you, you have just become this person's supplier. What's worse, your little white pills could end up at someone's pill party!

There are lots of teenagers that end up in Emergency Rooms because of this.

Remember that medicines are drugs and they become unsafe when they are not used as originally intended. The bottom line on this is, DON'T STORE YOUR MEDICATION IN YOUR BATHROOM MEDICINE CABINET!

So, where should you store them? In a locked box that you can then store in a cool dry place (or refrigerator, if that is what the manufacturer recommends).

This was not the reaction I was looking for!--
Author, Ms. Addie Venture

MY MEDICINE HAS MADE ME MORE ILL- NOW WHAT?

So you have done everything in your power to get better and you take a medication that causes an unbearable effect, what should you do? Who should you tell? Houston, we have a problem!

Depending on the severity of the reaction, do not be afraid to go to the emergency room! If you are having trouble breathing, go to the emergency room! If you are not sure if it could be serious or not, go to the emergency room! After you are properly treated, inform your prescriber of what happened and bring the discharge papers from the hospital with you.

Take a look at this information regarding allergic reactions. You may want to do it now, before you actually need it and you can always refer to it later:

http://www.aaaai.org/conditions-and-treatments/library/at-a-glance/medications-and-drug-allergic-reactions.aspx

For prescription and non prescription drugs, foods, nutritional supplements, biologicals (ex blood products),--combination products and cosmetics_ use MedWatch:

https://www.accessdata.fda.gov/scripts/medwatch/index.cfm?action=consumer.reporting1

for more information on this type of reporting, see:

https://www.accessdata.fda.gov/scripts/medwatch/index.cfm?action=reporting.home

For vaccines use VAERS (Vaccine Adverse Event Reporting System)

https://vaers.hhs.gov/esub/step1

DON'T POLLUTE OUR WATER

I can remember as a child being told to flush certain things. Even after graduating Pharmacy school in the early 1990's, I did not have a clear vision of what to do with unnecessary medications at home.

At work, that was easy because we had systems in place for that. We had a designated area for expired medications. We had procedures in place for excess controlled substances because of the specifics of the law governing these substances and their destruction. So I did not run into that problem at work.

But what do I tell someone who wants to properly dispose of their medications? That was a grey area back then (and it was not that long ago).

Fast forward to today, people are living longer, people who would have died of certain diseases because of medical advances aren't dying. There are so many treatments for diseases that were untreatable even just a few years ago. Cities are crowded (or is it just my city? Hmmm!). Many people are co-morbid (have more than one disease). Think about it, if everyone flushed their unused and expired medications, we would have a real problem!

What I would tell you to do is mostly what the FDA says:

- look for a DEA Drug Take Back Day in your area or go to their website, www. dea.gov for more information. Make sure that it is DEA sponsored! If you have controlled substances to get rid of make sure that you can bring them because, there must be law enforcement present in order for you to use this option...I say this because some drug take back days don't have the option for controlled substances to be left, so make sure you find out before you go. In my opinion the *DEA Drug Take Back Day* is the better option.
- mix your unused/unwanted medication with either used coffee grounds or kitty litter. This option is not fool proof. Drug

addicts are desperate folks, need I say more!

Take a look at this handout for more information...

http://www.takebackyourmeds.org/what-you-can-do/medicine-disposal-myths-and-facts

Mom! Steven took my diary and won't give it back!
---*Author, Steven's frustrated teenage sister*

THE ONE DIARY YOU SHOULD SHARE

If you are anywhere near my age, you know someone that has kept a diary. The contents of this diary were always of a personal nature. Because of this, diaries became hot commodities used to fulfill the pranks of little brothers and others that had the nefarious intent of blackmail on their minds.

It does not matter if you are male or female, young or old, I want you to keep a diary! This diary is one that you will share. Ideally, you will give one copy to someone that you trust and you will keep the other copy on your person (in your wallet or your phone, whichever is more convenient for you). The diary that you will keep is a medication diary.

Your medication diary is very similar to the profile that your Pharmacist has on file about you. You need to have a record of your medications. It should be updated every time you have a medication added, changed or discontinued. You should have one for each member of your family.

Why? Well. friend, you never know when it will happen, where it will happen or how it will happen but know that it will happen and if it hasn't happened yet, you are probably overdue! The "it" that I am talking about is the trip to the emergency room!

This is the place where they will ask about your medications. The EMTs will also request this information in the ambulance. Instead of trying to recall names that you cannot pronounce and dosages and strengths that you can't remember, why not have it written down or have it in your phone? Wouldn't that make things a lot easier?

Let me tell you that a great part of my experience has been in the hospital setting and most hospitals will not let a patient take their own medication in their facility. Why is this? Well because, it is a huge liability for them, there are just too many unknowns... has the medication been stored properly? has anyone switched the medication out of the bottle? how old is that tablet (has the medication expired)? The litany of questions goes on and on and on.

In some hospitals, the medication that a patient comes in with is confiscated, itemized and sent to the pharmacy to be stored. In some hospitals, the medication is confiscated and given to a family member to take home.

So back to the medication diary, you are going to list every prescription drug, every non prescription drug, every supplement, etc. It does not matter whether you take the medicine orally, by injection, place it on the skin, etc...you will list it all!

Additionally, you will list what time of day you take each medicine, the strength of your medicine, the doctor who prescribed your medicine, etc. You will list your known allergies. You see, these are the things that medical practitioners will need to know about you and your therapy! In an emergency situation, every second counts!

For an example of this medication diary, you can download this link:

https://onedrive.live.com/redir?resid=97440F8F 2BA0878D!608&authkey=!AMSOc6_mtNPrRWI& ithint=file%2cdocx

About the Author

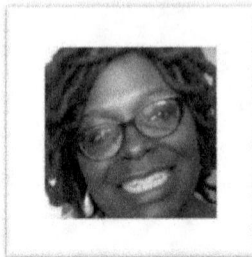

Vanessa_LeSure-Walker is a Pharmacist with over 17 years of experience behind the counter. She has worked in both Hospital and Retail Pharmacy environments. She has worked for over 11 years to help Pharmacy Technicians become certified.

She is the Founder of The APhTI Project and thus has taken on two very important missions. The first is to help Pharmacy Technicians achieve their personal best. She believes that in order for technicians to master all of pharmacy's moving parts, they have to be coached into it.

The other is to bring the topic of Medication Safety to the forefront of education. She believes herself to be a Medication Safety Advocate and encourages patients and caregivers to learn more about the medications that they take and/or administer. Vanessa speaks regularly on this topic and other topics that she is passionate about.

She is also the author of Fundamental Formulas for Pharmacy Technicians which will be released later in 2015. She resides in the New York City area with her husband and two children.

You can reach Vanessa at vw@aphti.com. Her social media information is as follows:

Vanessa Walker RPh
Facebook: facebook.com/theaphtiproject
Blog: theaphtiproject.blogspot.com
Youtube: http://bit.ly/16JGZtq
LinkedIn:
https://www.linkedin.com/in/vanessalesurewalk
er

If you are interested in joining my mailing list or in obtaining a medication storage box with a lock for your household or for travel purposes, you can email info@aphti.com with your contact information(email address and phone number) and someone from my office will get back to you.

Now that you have this information, what are the things that you will do differently regarding your medications?

_____

_____

_____

_____

_____

_____

_____

_____

_____

_____

_____

_____

www.ingramcontent.com/pod-product-compliance
Lightning Source LLC
Chambersburg PA
CBHW070933180526
45168CB00003B/1062